Yoga and How to Stay Stress-Less:

Alternative therapy approaches

Yoga Volume # 3

By Doris Richardson- Edsell

Copyright by Doris Richardson-Edsell, June 2014

Yoga photos by Sarah Grace

Table of Contents

About the Author: Doris Richardson-Edsell is registered nurse, yoga teacher, mother and grandmother who has authored 19 books on Amazon. She writes daily on her website Body Mind Health www.body-mindhealth.com Doris is a strong advocate for those who have difficulties with emotions, and her goal is to bring wellness in mind, body and spirit to everyone who seeks to balance their lives.

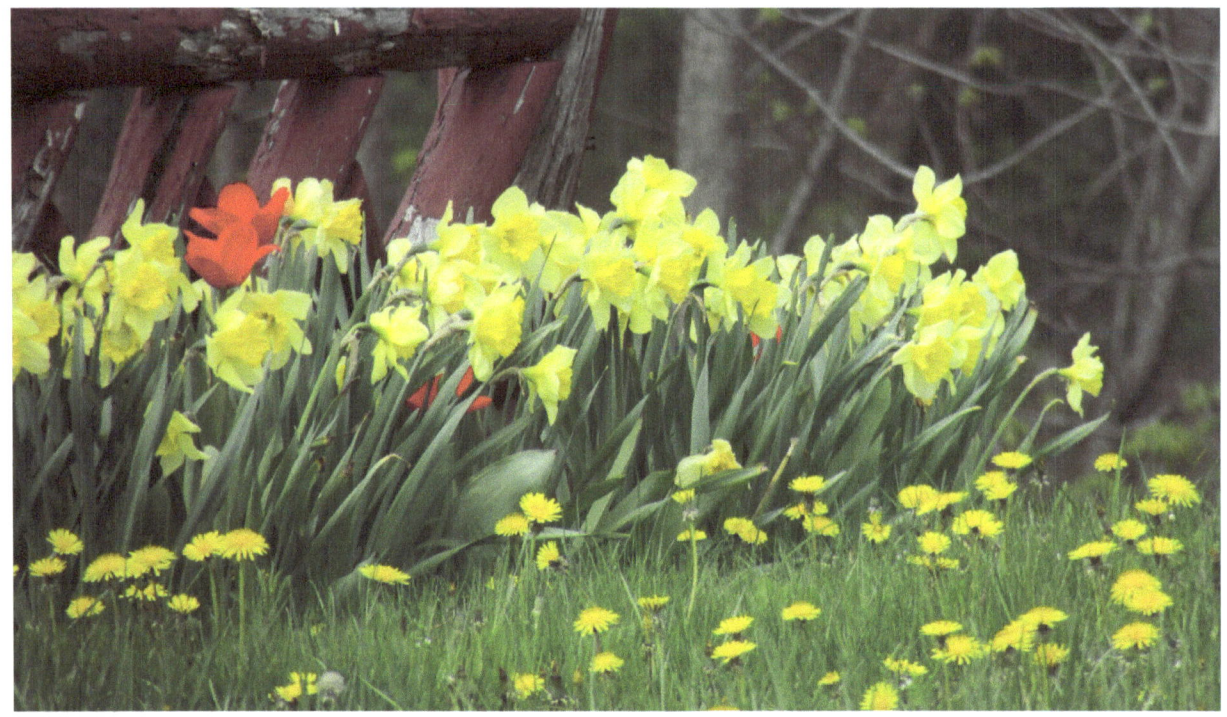

Flowers strive for wellness, bending their beauty toward the sunshine; and weeds too are sturdy and hard to get rid of

I believe that everyone wants to be well in mind, body and spirit and that is why I write every day to speak on how to stay healthy.

You have to work at it; different modalities can help you move toward a healthy living goal in life.

Why should you practice yoga?

Yoga has attracted much attention in the past few years because it has helped so very many people to heal in mind, body and spirit, but there are other Eastern modalities that you can add to your yoga practice such as acupressure and tapping points, Qigong, Reiki and tai chi to name a few. Many of these healing activities focus on moving energy throughout your body so that you can heal and they honor your body by helping you to take better care of yourself through breathing better, slowing things down and remembering that life is as it should be, one beautiful moment after another.

Aging and your health

Did you know that as you age, you require less food?

If you are an active older person you may need to make sure that you do not cut back on necessary nutrients because you may eat less now. And as the body ages it is less likely to be able to process heavy food such as creamy mixtures or even meats that can be inflammatory such as red meat. You may find that you are looking for alternatives to meat protein; grains and beans can be a good choice for you; they are easier on your digestive system.

Mind Power

As you age you may need to take a look at how to nourish you mind with inspirational and positive focused readings which can help you to keep your *mind power* strong.

Nourishing the Spirit

As you learn the different alternative modalities such as yoga, you will begin to nourish your spiritual growth too. Learning how to slow down the breath and just breathe; learning how important meditative practice can be to your health and learning how stillness, flexibility and balance can also add to your continuing wellness in mind, body and spirit.

Breathe in and Breathe Out

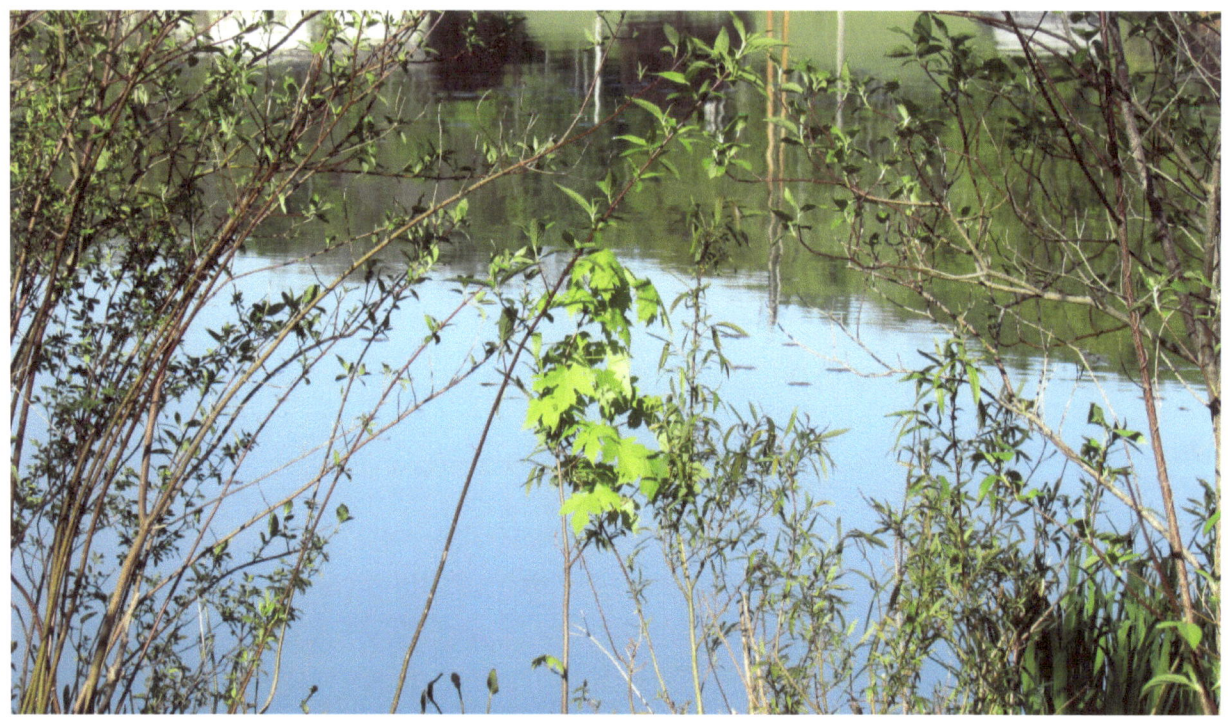

Take a break and just gaze at the wonder of nature. It slows you down, and you can capture peace for a moment in time

Slow Down, you move too fast!

There is so much information on the fact that you can slow just about everything down just by learning how to breathe better. Slowing down the rhythm of your breath can be so very helpful in many situations.

When it comes to stressful times, just being able to gather yourself, still, quiet and centered can be so very helpful.

These easy breathing techniques should be taught to very young children, and may even prevent such ailments as asthma because one learns how to slow down the breath and stay calm even when your body may be saying otherwise. Placing ones hands at your heart center and placing some pressure on the breastbone has also been found to help slow down the breath.

Practicing a Simple Breathing Technique

Practice is the best way to start breathing techniques. Breathe in through your nose for the count of 5, very slowly, and watch your belly bellow out. Next hold your breath for a second before exhaling for a count of 7, watching you stomach suck in. Do this a few times a day and you will notice the difference.

A Relaxation Mode

Lying down is the best way to practice relaxation. Laying on you back, hands are palms up on the side of your body. Legs spread out a bit with your feet moving outward. Put your hands on your belly and feel your belly rise with each soft and slow breath.

And if you want a more special moment, put on some soft music while you practice your breathing.

Stress

If you have a stressful job, or feel stressed out, breathing practice can not only slow you down, it may save your life. With this new found ability to self- soothe, you will be calmer and more able to face the world and life's daily difficulties.

Moments

Practice moment to moment mindfulness. You do not have to focus on the future happenings, or what has happened in the past. Be with your moment right now, without distractions. Allow the negative to just flow out of you, and embrace each positive moment in time.

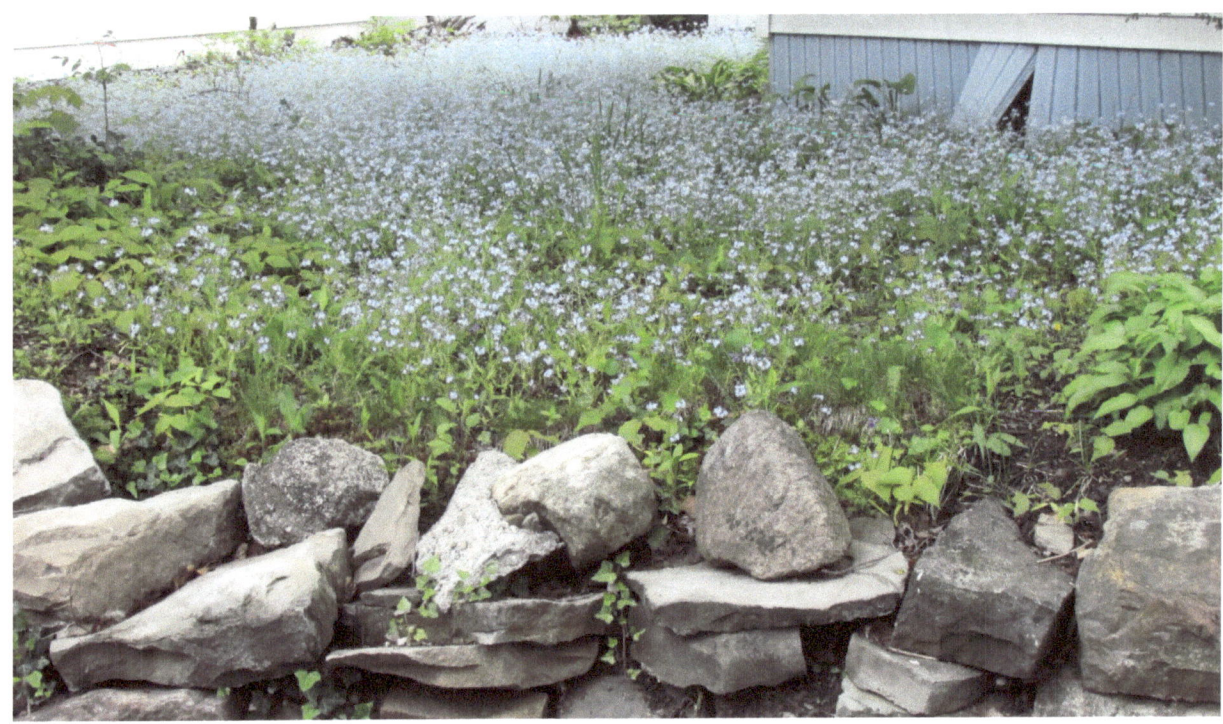

Capture moments of blue bliss

Just Be

I have been trying for years to become *de-stressed.*

There are many kinds of remedies, but I feel that the best ones are those that work for you. Your own special way of staying calm and centered in your daily life can be a life saver for you someday. In this hectic world, people just seem to strive on staying busy and creating their own stress!

My Special Moments are in Meditation

I have been meditating for a few years, and it helps me, but it is definitely a skill that one has to develop especially if you are fidgety. People who have a hard time sitting still really have a difficult time with learning to meditate or just plain relax!

If you have been trying meditation for a long time, and it does not seem to work for you, then it is time to *switch it up*. You may want to try relaxation instead. Just lying down with some special music to ponder on is a good way.
And what works for you right now may not work in the future, therefore, to become *stress-less,* you need a tool box of things to do and try.
For example, when I feel that I am going to have a rough day, I start it out with some sort of yoga routine. It might just be a few minutes of downward facing dog pose so that I get some blood to my brain, or it may be just listening to some soft music that helps me to feel calmer. Or just being quiet. Sometimes when I am driving, I turn off the radio just to concentrate on one thing- my driving!

Accepting the Way Things Are

Accept that your life will have some ups and downs. Try your best to let them mostly be ups! Manage yourself carefully so that you do not have to rush off somewhere. Give yourself enough time to get where you need to go. Stop the rushed living and find pleasure in daily activities.

The world is a beautiful place; start to enjoy it with some peace in your life. Make every single moment count.

Caught up in the moment

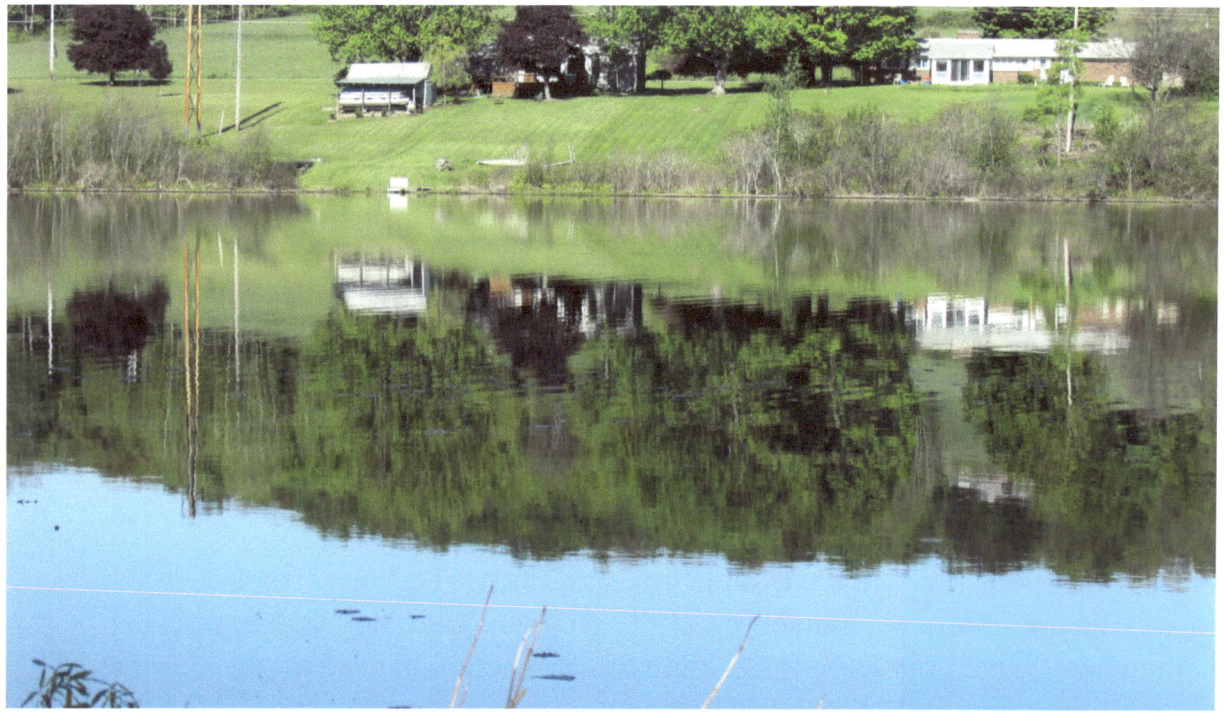

Find your bliss in some water scenes. Reflecting a positive moment in time

When I was a child, an art teacher taught me about how difficult it is to paint water scenes because you may have to paint a reflection and it has to be perfect because in nature there is perfection, unlike the painter's hand.

Ever since I studied art, I have been amazed by all kind of natural beauty. Reflection can cause our eyes to see the same pattern upside down. And what a joy it is to see a wonderful picture made by nature and reflecting water.

Colorless wonders

When you look at something that is colorless like rocks and stones, you still see patterns and shapes that form a beautiful picture, and the slight colors forming throughout, fossils of lost bugs, or green moss on the edges.

Even stones piled up neatly, or not so neatly, can be beautiful because each one is different shape and size just like humans are. We are all different, and because of these differences, we are unique.

One rock after another, piled high

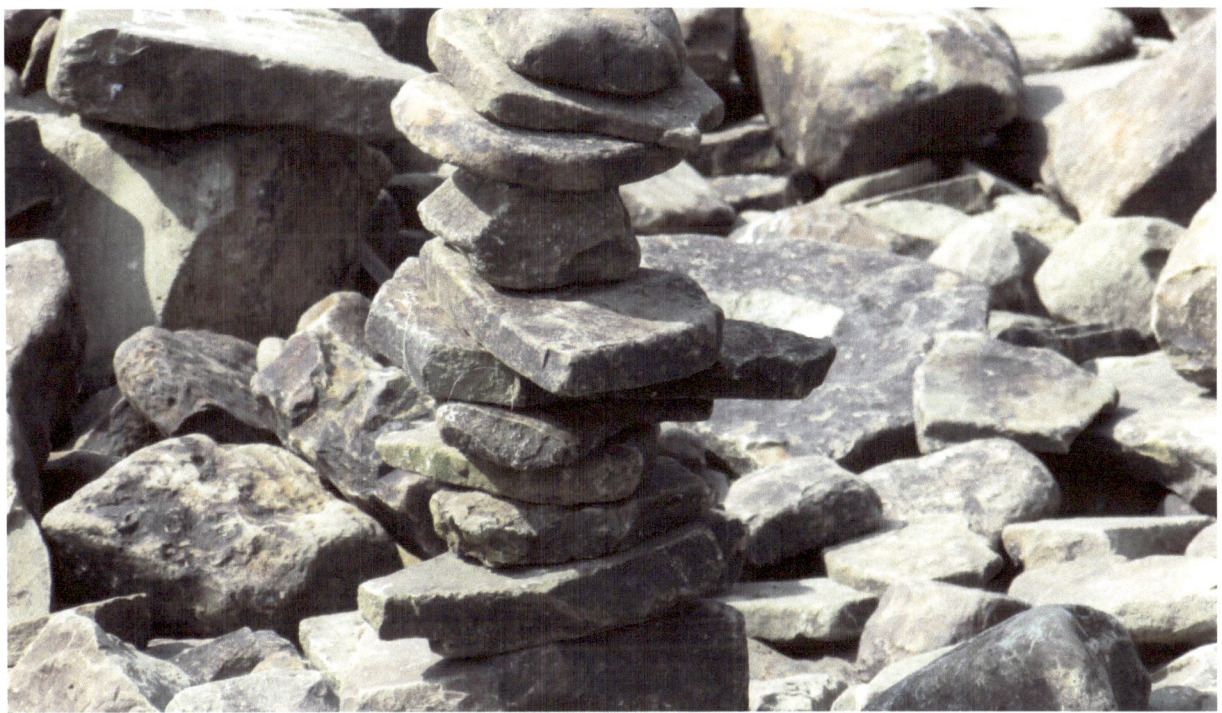

You can be like the piles of rock with your thoughts. Sometimes you cannot stop yourself from thinking those bad things over and over again and they begin to pile up. Maybe you should get caught up in the beauty of things just the way they are and how each one is an individual creation, worn out by a lake nearby.

Caught in the moment of living life

I have to admit that sometimes I get caught up in life; caught in the moment of negative thinking that just makes me feel bad. When this happens, the first thing that I try to do is take a walk and clear those thoughts.

Happiness

You need to stop… and think about where you are going. Do you want to be a happier person?

If you want happiness, you have to find a path toward being more positive.

If you are caught up in life, and in the fast lane, this can put damper on your mental health, your spirit and your physical well-being.

Anger and health

I know that when I am angry about something, or just thinking bad thoughts, I often turn to some bad past behaviors such as eating too much; and then I feel worse about myself and my situation. Low self-esteem seems to be the consequence for many people who *swim* in bad thoughts.

That is why it is so important to find good alternatives that may help you to think better about yourself and the good, bad and ugly things that happen to everyone.
Walking and thinking better thoughts really helps me to be more centered and in touch with myself.

What kinds of things do you do to get out of your funk?

How do you put more joy into your life so that you are happier and content?

Journaling you way toward a happier you

Start a journal and write down some positive affirmations about yourself.
Examples: I feel confident in my ability to bring joy and happiness into my life.
When I look in the mirror, I see a positive person who is smiling and having fun in life's journey!
When I have bad thought, I will just let it pass like the wind has come under it to take it away.

Yoga and Yin Asanas: Helping with Flexibility

A new flexible you

There are theories on different types of exercise that help with flexibility and the restoration of some worn out parts.

The first part that seems to go are the hips, and many people who teach on yoga believe that you can restore or recondition some of what ails you.
Bernie Clark is his book on yoga entitled: *The Complete Guide to Yin Yoga* speaks on the best asanas (poses) that can help with bringing some of your parts back into alignment.

Some of the poses include dragon for stretching both the groin and hips, shoelace, pigeon, child's pose and melting heart all open up the hips, allowing for more flexible hips.

When you meditate softly in the poses below, you can feel the stretch that helps you get your hips back into shape. I like to start out with shoe lace and then move into pigeon and finally wide-legged child's pose, and then I slide up into melting heart.

Remember that there is no pain, numbness or tingling in these exercises; you should feel stretching, and it should be soothing; if not, come out of the pose and go into a less stressful pose such as child's pose.

Mending the Hips

When you start out your yoga practice it is a good idea to do the yin poses (softer, longer holding poses) first, and then move into the yang flows later in your practice.

Learning how to do shoelace is a good first start. Here is a picture of the pose. Remember that this pose may take some time for you to be completely flexible in; you may have to start with half a lace.

Shoelace

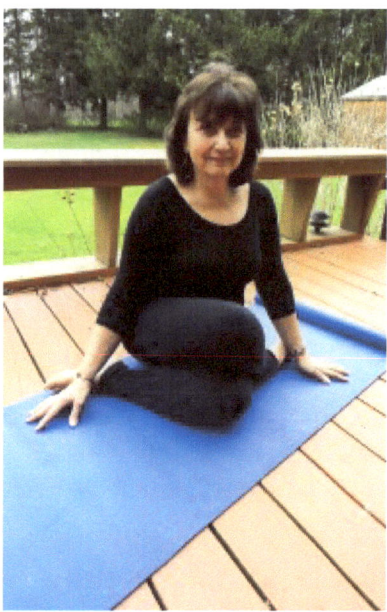

Shoelace helps with the hips. If you can stay in this pose for about 3-5 minutes each side, you will have a nice beginning to your yin practice.

Another pose that helps with your hips is Pigeon. When you hold in pigeon pose for about 3-5 minutes each side, you can feel your hips move into a good place.

Pigeon

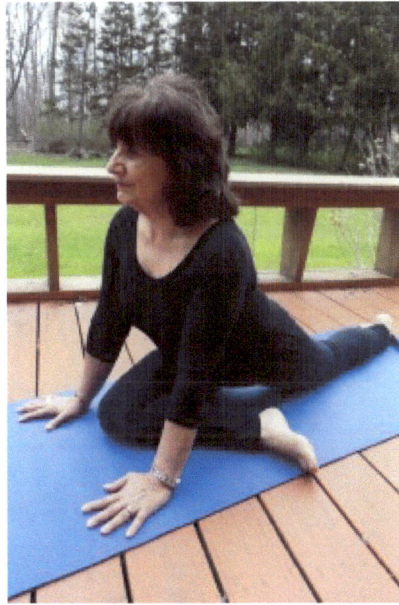

Start out in an upward pigeon like shown, and then slide hands forward and head down into full pigeon pose.

Another deeper pose that helps with the hips is called Dragon. Dragon opens up the hips and the groin. If you have knee issues, you may want to place some padding under your knee that is in the back in both Pigeon and Dragon.

Here is a picture of Dragon- Side View

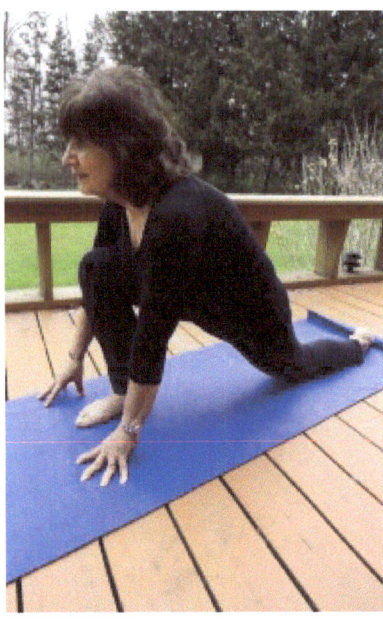

Dragon Front View

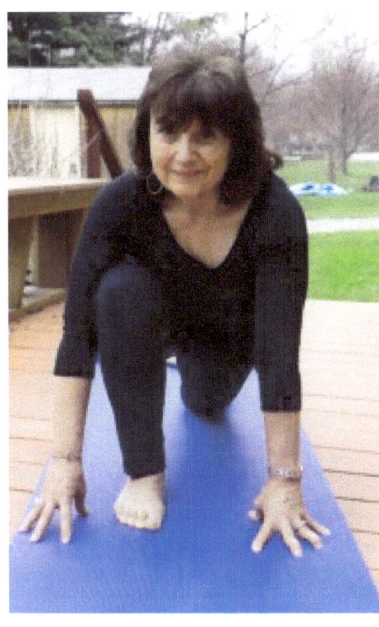

In yin poses, staying in the pose; resolving to stay still and feeling the meditative way, anchors you into the asanas; allowing for you to find ways to reach closer to the floor with each practice.

Counter-pose

After you do both Pigeon and Dragon, or in between each one, you may want to do a counter- pose to help relax the muscles and joints that are working hard. Child's pose is the asana that works for these strong yin poses. And wide legged child's pose with the arms up sliding across the mat and just the forehead touching the floor along with your big toes touching softly in the back. Here is a picture.

Child's Pose/ Melting heart.

After about 5 minutes of child's pose, slowly come out of the pose into melting heart. All you have to do is raise your but in the air, keeping your forehead down and arms stretched out as in the picture. And when you raise your buttocks in the air, your heart center sinks down (that is why it is called melting heart).

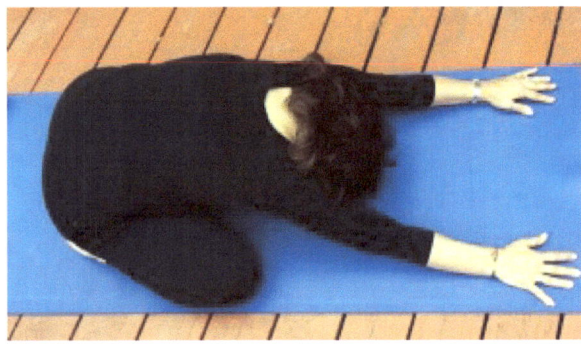

The straddle pose is a nice opener of the groin and hips, allowing for you to be upside down. As long as you do not have difficulties with high blood pressure, being upside down is a great thing for your entire body, allowing blood flow throughout.

Straddle Pose with assistance of a yoga block: Flexible people can do this pose with their head reaching the floor. Notice how I have my elbows pushing against the fatty cushions of my knees for extra stability.

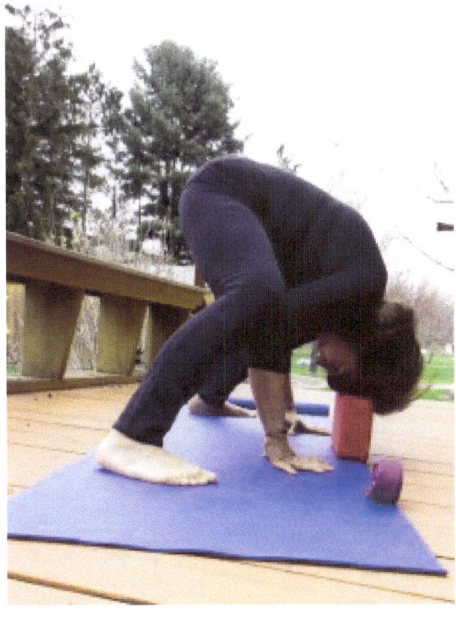

A deep pose for your legs, groin and hips. Straddle can help you with blood flow

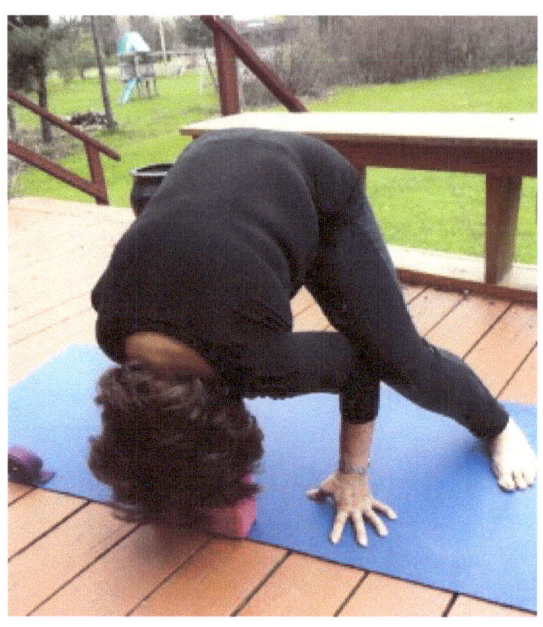

Different angle to look at the straddle pose

Many people have different levels of flexibility with straddle. Some can stretch their legs out very wide. (I am a bit limited with my straddle!)

Learning how to be more flexible especially in the hip and groin areas can help you later on in life when you may have some difficulties with you hip joints or knees, and yin yoga can help because when your hips get back in place so do your knees.

The practice of yin yoga also helps with meditation. When you *grow your practice*; learning to hold in the pose for more than just a few minutes; your flexibility and balance grow with you. Many people explore yoga to the extent of holding some yin poses for up to 15 minutes; the original intention of yoga was learning how to hold in poses for long times, preparing oneself for the deeper practice of meditation. The poses were considered a step toward learning how to just be within oneself; meditatively; with the spirit. I have found the most useful poses for development in the flexibility of the hips is Pigeon and Child's pose. Just moving from one to the other can really give you a good yin workout.

Ideas for yin poses: Clark, B (2011). *The Complete Guide to Yin Yoga.* White Cloud Press. Ashland, Oregon

Solutions for Stressful Times

Abstract art is the best because you do not have to please the eye of the beholder; they can imagine whatever they want to.

Photo: Taken at Sculpture Park, NY

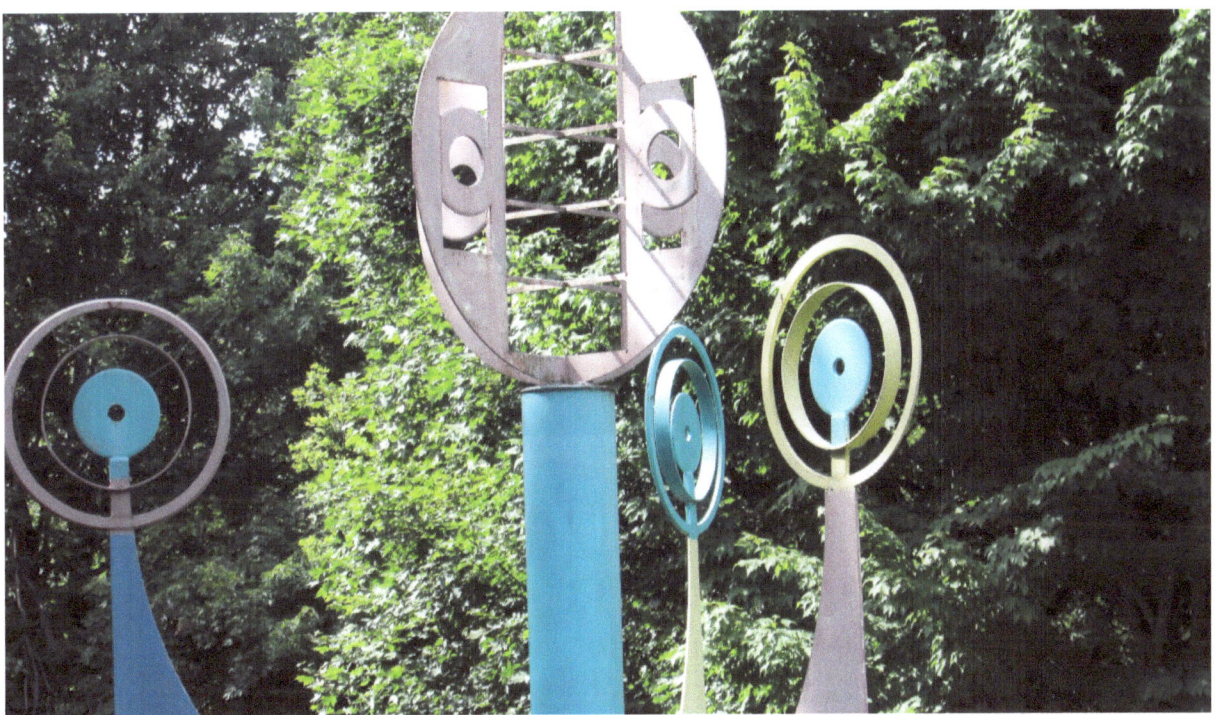

Resiliency: Some people are more resilient than others.

If you grow up in an environment of nurturing and kindness, you will probably be more resilient than most. If you grow up in a confusing, chaotic home, you may not be sure of yourself and your potential to grow and develop into a productive, loving person.

Can you re- balance yourself?

Dr. James Rouse who wrote *Health Solutions for Stress Relief and how to re-balance your natural stress-resilient body chemistry* believes that you can become more resilient to the stress in life by practicing alternative therapies such as yoga.

Be on alert and combat the stressful times by eating healthy foods

Your body is on alert from what your mind is telling it. When bad things happen, or you just feel overwhelmed by too many tasks, your body gets the hint and goes on overdrive. You have to begin to see the connection between your body, mind and spirit to help yourself out of stressful times. You may even have to take a look at your diet, and eat some stress reducing recipes.

Let's start with the diet. Diet can play a major role in stress reduction just as exercise does, so no matter how much yoga or running you may do, if you do not change to more nutritious foods and watch your sugar, you may still have problems with the stress in your life.

The local markets

Try your best to seek out fresh foods from your local farmers. Organics are a bit more expensive, but there is no greater expense in life than poor health and wellness.

Find foods that can manage your blood sugar, (such as fiber foods), calm inflammation (that may mean staying away from red meat and deep fried foods) and can help you reach your weight loss goals.

Everything in life is about balance, therefore, you need to balance through portion control, eating lots of fruits and veggies and making healthy choices every single day!

Eating with Consciousness

Food serves a purpose in helping you to stay healthy and you should respect it. A mindful approach to eating is essential for the spirit. Think about your food when you sit down to eat, and try your best to eat slowly, tasting every bite of food.

Combining foods

Some foods combine well while others do not

The goal is to aim for some rich protein products such as lean turkey, tofu or cottage cheese, and adding some whole grains. In order for your body to accept the protein, and make it available to the brain, protein needs to be combined with complex carbohydrates such as brown rice or whole-grains.

Energy and sustaining satisfaction throughout the day

By combining rich proteins with complex carbohydrates, you will begin to enjoy more energy in your day.

Complex carbs also supply glucose for the brain.

Your Eating Plan for Reducing Stress

Focus on enjoyment! Reinforce some healthy, glucose-friendly whole grains, fruits and veggies. Most high- glycemic foods are refined. For example: Foods made with white flour spike your blood sugar and fail to provide your body with essential vitamins and minerals. Stay away from pasta, breads other foods made with white flour.

On the other hand, foods that are low in the glycemic index tend to be nutrient dense, boost your energy and even boost your metabolism. Such foods like healthy grains (quinoa, amaranth, barley, whole grain wheat berries) can last a long time in your body, creating satiety.

Some veggies

Arame seaweed- rich in minerals and B vitamins

Broccoli- the super veggie that is high in antioxidants

Cabbage- another superfood linked to cancer prevention

Carrots- beta-carotene helps the body disarm destructive compounds that attack cells

Celery- In Chinese medicine it is used to treat high blood pressure, along with being low in sugar

Some Fruits

Apples are number one! Rich in fiber, one apple has as much fiber as about 10 small salads

Bananas rich in tryptophan and potassium. A sliced banana on toast with some peanut butter can support the neurotransmitters that encourage sleep and tranquility

Blueberries- powerful antioxidants provide brain and memory support

Dates- High in fiber

Grapefruit- Good source of Vitamin C and pectin. They are very healthy for the digestive tract.

Lemons- Rich in Vitamin C. they are a great immunity booster. As an internal cleanser- lemon with some water in the morning can acts as an internal cleanser

Oranges- Rich in Vitamin C and have high levels of hesperidin, a flavonoid that fights cancer and heart disease

Strawberries- high in antioxidants, especially the one called ellogic acid which is believed to be a great inhibitor of cancer

Grains and Legumes

Brown rice is a great source of insoluble fiber. Brown rice can actually pick up cholesterol and pull it right out as it moves through the body. Also is great for bowel regularity and is rich in manganese an important mineral for bone health and blood sugar regulation

Lentils- Power-packed with folate, magnesium and fiber

Oats- Lower blood cholesterol and promotes heart health. Eat oats for magnesium, B vitamins and tryptophan, and because oats are a complex carbohydrate, you can get the benefits of tryptophan by eating them alone.

Whole grains – amaranth, kamut, millet, quinoa and wheat: Whole grains also include whole grains in bread, cereals, muffins, wheat bran and wheat germ

Dairy, including Almond and Soy Milk

Milk is a stress reduction tool, rich in tryptophan and calcium

Soy and almond milk: high in calcium and provides anti-inflammatory benefits

Tofu- High in calcium

Yogurt (soy and dairy), mozzarella cheese and cottage cheese- high in tryptophan and calcium

Fish

Halibut, salmon and mackerel are all a great source of omega-3 fatty acids

Chicken and turkey- good sources of tryptophan which is a building block of serotonin and melatonin, a supporter of brain functioning and sleep aid!

Eggs are rich in omega-3 fatty acids and a good source of tryptophan. And the protein in eggs can help keep blood sugar stable

Lean Beef- provides for Vitamin B 3

Almonds and almond butter- improves cholesterol

Flaxseed- rich in omega-3 providing for the heart and can prevent cancer

Hazelnuts- rich in omega-3 and helps with lowering cholesterol

Olive oil- Rich in monounsaturated fats

Peanuts and Cashews- peanuts are high in tryptophan and cashews rich in monounsaturated (beneficial fats)

Pumpkin Seeds- mineral dense and rich in zinc and magnesium. Particularly good for stress reduction and boosting the immune system along with heart health

Taken in part from: Rouse, J. (2003) *Health Solutions for Stress Relief.* Rodale press at www. rodale.com

You are Still There

You can run away from things but deep inside you are still there

If any emotion overcomes you because you allow it to, you are there, on your own; helping yourself, or not helping. Emotions can be wonderful; they show people how much you care, but difficult emotions such as sadness or anger can stay with you too long and you may need to take a deeper look at yourself; centering on the positive whenever you can. There is much positive to look at in the world, and angry words, feelings or thoughts need to be put aside.

Centering

Staying in the center is where I want to be. No matter what happens, I want to be alright; not overly happy or sad. It seems like a reasonable request of my internal being because I have been around for many years, and I know that being on either side is overwhelming, even if it is happiness. There has to be a break in the stream of any type of emotion, whether it is good or bad.

You can try to hide behind some things in life, but you are still there

It does not matter where you are physically; you can run away from things, but there you are inside; spirit and emotions, clinging to you wherever you go.

You are always there, deep inside yourself

You are there in mind, body and spirit even when you are trying to move away from some things that may be bothering you. Those bad thoughts do not go away left untended or ignored; (out of sight is not always out of mind).

You carry everything with you like a big blue, yellow and green tapestry bag filled with the good, bad, and ugly things; even if you think that you have put them in the past.

Resolution

You may need to resolve some of your issues that are of concern, because tucking them away, even if you do it neatly, does not work; it is still there unsolved, unresolved, waiting for you to work on them.

Your spirit may tell you to wake up and look at yourself. Your mind may do the same with some emotional outbursts that you may not like, or the inability to feel the pain.

Talking to others may help; even a good counselor can help, but you need to do the work.

You cannot keep moving along hiding from whatever it is that makes you feel too sad, angry or depressed to express.

My Hidden Thoughts

For many years I was good at hiding from bad things; people thought that I was doing well; they did not know about my true feelings because I did not speak; believing that eventually things would resolve unattended.

What happened is what happens to any untended garden; it over grows, looks terrible and then there is so much work to do on it that you may not know where to begin, so you give up and plow it over.

In life, I cannot plow anything over; but I am beginning to see that many things just don't matter; and with that said, I need to do the hard work of bringing things into harmony for myself because I only have one life and I want the rest of it to be as happy as possible.

Therapeutic Movements

When I think of movement, I think of running, jumping or walking, but slow therapeutic movements are something that can be healing. And you do not have to be an expert; you can even make up your own movements that guide you toward health and wellness; spiritual movement that are slow and purposeful. Eastern philosophy seems to have many modalities that heal the body; acupressure points and tapping, Qigong and Tai Chi just to name a few.

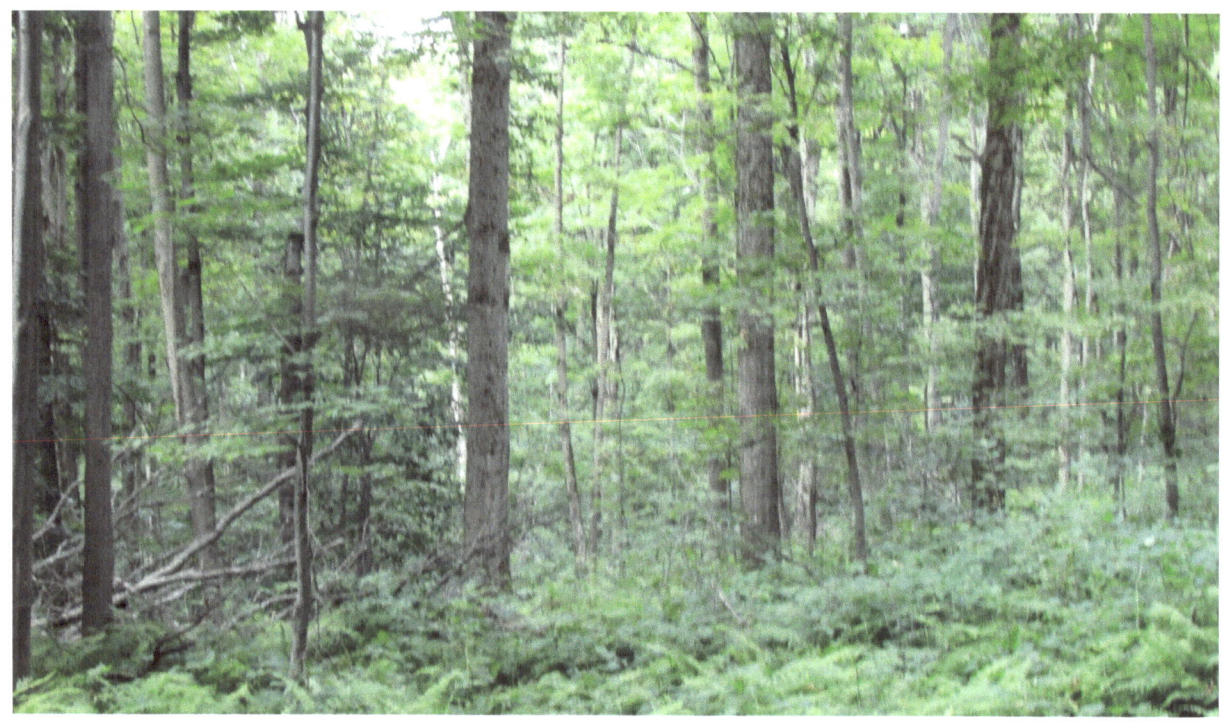

Walking slowly down the path near my home can be therapeutic to my mind, body and soul

Rubbing and Tapping

Easterners believe in rubbing the feet, hands and ears as ways to move energy throughout the body. During my yoga classes, I teach a type of energy release along with acupressure points and tapping on various parts of the body such as the top of the head, between the nose, the cheekbones, temples and all the way down the body.

I speak on yoga quite frequently but there are other modalities that can be helpful in a quest toward wellness.

Qigong

Another modality is Qigong, a healing energy *Qi* that helps keep you centered and focused with your breath and energy centers like yoga.

Qigong like Yoga and Reiki centers on learning stillness, slowing the breath, restoring health, and promoting well-being.

Stuck energy centers

Practitioners of Qigong feel that you may have stuck energy in the body that needs to be released and then healing can occur. Michael Tse in his book *Qigong for Health and Vitality* speaks on this energy release from simple exercises that generate internal energy.

By practicing Qigong you are allowing your Qi (energy) to strengthen your internal being, promoting stillness and harmony in mind, body and soul. When you develop your Qi through Qigong, your body becomes balanced; bringing your body to a point between consciousness and unconsciousness, where you are neither awake nor asleep. With the movement; your whole body comes to a balanced state and relaxes. This is where you can begin to forget about everything and just be.

Your body becomes quiet and you do not notice your breathing. Doing Qigong exercises can optimize the power of your brain and improve your memory. And when you begin a practice of Qigong you become calm, relaxed and open due to the energy releasing Qi.

Stuck Energy Center thoughts from- Tse, M. (1996) *Qigong for health and vitality.* New York, NY. St. Martin's Griffin

Memories that Change

Your mind keeps memories sacredly tucked away, and for some memories, that is a blessing

There are different parts in your brain for the good, bad and ugly things in life. Some great memories are as clear as the moment they happened, and very accurate; other memories may be unclear because you really do not want to remember them; they are usually the bad ones.

I would like to believe that wherever I am down the path of life; memories are good

And then there are the unclear ones; these are the memories that grow into different things completely; you change them on a daily basis to fit your needs; sort of like changing your mood from a bad one to a good mood. Emotional memories that bring about sadness, happiness, elation or even a smile are the ones that can change a lot.

Lost Memories can be found: Preserving the Memory and then letting it go

You may have had some hard times with someone, got divorced or just went your separate ways, and then the memories in your mind changed. At first you may remember only the bad memories and then all of a sudden some of the good ones start to pop into your head when you are triggered by something such as seeing an object that person had given to you as a gift that you had long forgotten.

Symbols of the past

I have a chair that someone had given me as a birthday gift and I cannot remember the year but I remember being in the antique store somewhere in the Southern part of New York. I loved that wonderful piece; a colorful tapestry rocker that captured my heart. And last week I decided it was so special that I needed to pass it along to my daughter and then to my granddaughter when she turns 30. I may be here only in spirit when the gift gets passed along, but I wanted to be the one to make sure that this special gift gets *re-gifted* in a special way.

On getting older

As you get older, you may want to preserve some of the good things about your past; take a look back and see what you can pass along. It does not have to be a material thing; passing along some good advice is also a sound gift.

Whatever it is, it is a good thing to re-capture some good out of some bad times. And this re-capturing seems to grow stronger as you move toward spiritual living. If you believe in life after death, you may want to get your spiritual inner being ready for the journey!

The Good in everything

I would like to believe it is a fact that there is good in everything that happens to you, even in the worst of times. My past relationships were not as good as I wanted them to be, and because of that, they ended. I kept on looking for something better in life, and finally in my 50's I found that I am the person who decides how good I feel, and I can make almost every situation in life a better one.

Healing those bad feelings

If you still find it hard to find some good in some of the bad things that have happened to you; keep walking down that road and find the place in your head where everything is in place.

Life is like a puzzle with many pieces that fall out of place, and it may take some time to put the puzzle together, especially if it is a difficult one.

My mom loved puzzles; she kept them out on a card table for months putting them together, and when she was done, she immediately started another. I asked her, "Why don't you take a break from puzzles?" and mom said," You have to keep your mind fresh with new thoughts to get your through the day."

When you reminisce on the past, change your thought process to a different way of seeing things; just like the puzzle or a long road without an end, life can have unusual twists and turns right ahead where you can change your mind about anything.

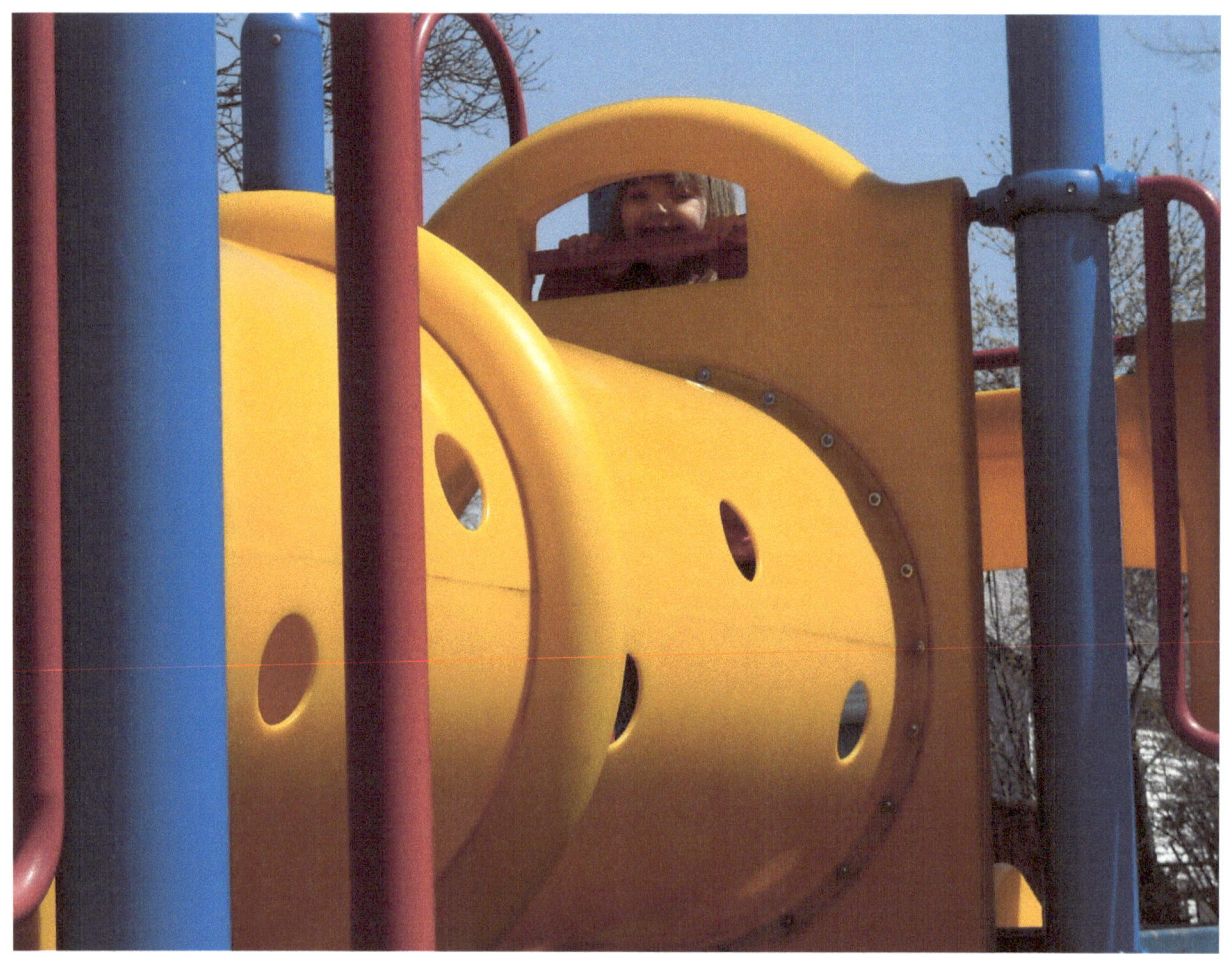

Remember when you were a child and you had purity of thought?
Children may not always be accurate with their interpretation of what adults
are saying or doing, but they are truthful

Stop Stealing Energy from Yourself

Every single time that you do something that is stressful or agonizing, think about how it is stealing from you and your life and how you may need to change.

Stealing takes away your energy and you may be unable to focus on anything because you have given your peace away.

Yoga Helps

In yoga, the practice of helping yourself before you can help others is very clearly stated in Alice Christensen's book, *Yoga of the Heart.* You have to make your life full and whole before you can help others do the same. In the springtime, you may need to clear out some of the things in life that are stealing from you. Many people keep things they do not need and if you have a lot of extra things, find ways to give them away or throw them out if they are of no use to anyone.

Concentration

Stealing from yourself can manifest in many ways such as not being able to concentrate because your internal robbers such as your *worry center* may take over your inner being. You may have to find ways to honor yourself with quiet, loving activities that do not steal from you, but add to your life. Gardening is an example. Look at what can be done when you tend to your garden well.

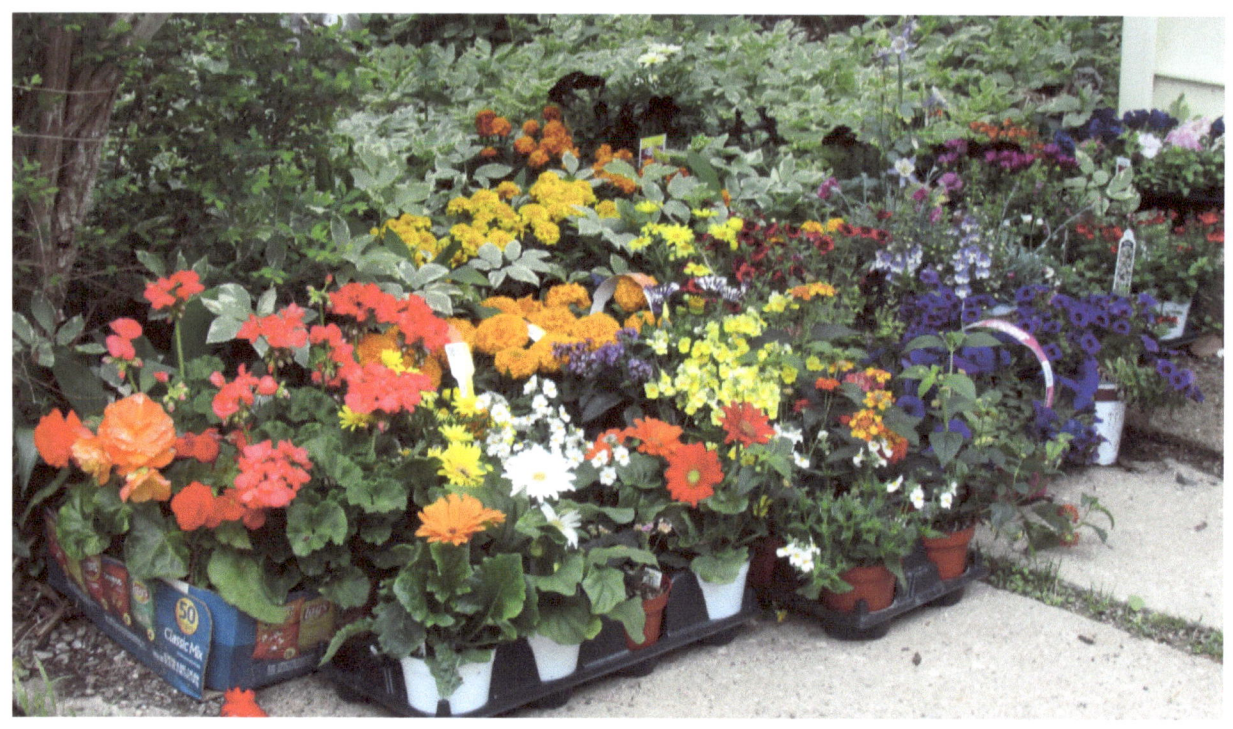

A true gardener wants their garden of life to be colorful and lovingly tended to

Watch yourself and guide your internal spirit toward preserving energy that can be used in activities that make you smile.

It will be time soon to get your flowers blooming, and garden activities can mellow your soul.

Your Spirit

Take time today to visit your spirit inside of you, the one who sends you messages telling you how important it is to take care of yourself. Choose a color today that makes your smile. When I want to feel good, I bring yellow and pinks into my life and take a walk, listening to nature at its best. Yellow is the color of sunshine, bringing you positive rays of energy.

Ideas on not stealing, ethical principles section: Christiansen, A. (1998) *Yoga of the Heart.* American Yoga Association. NY. NY Rodale Press

Is Yoga For You?

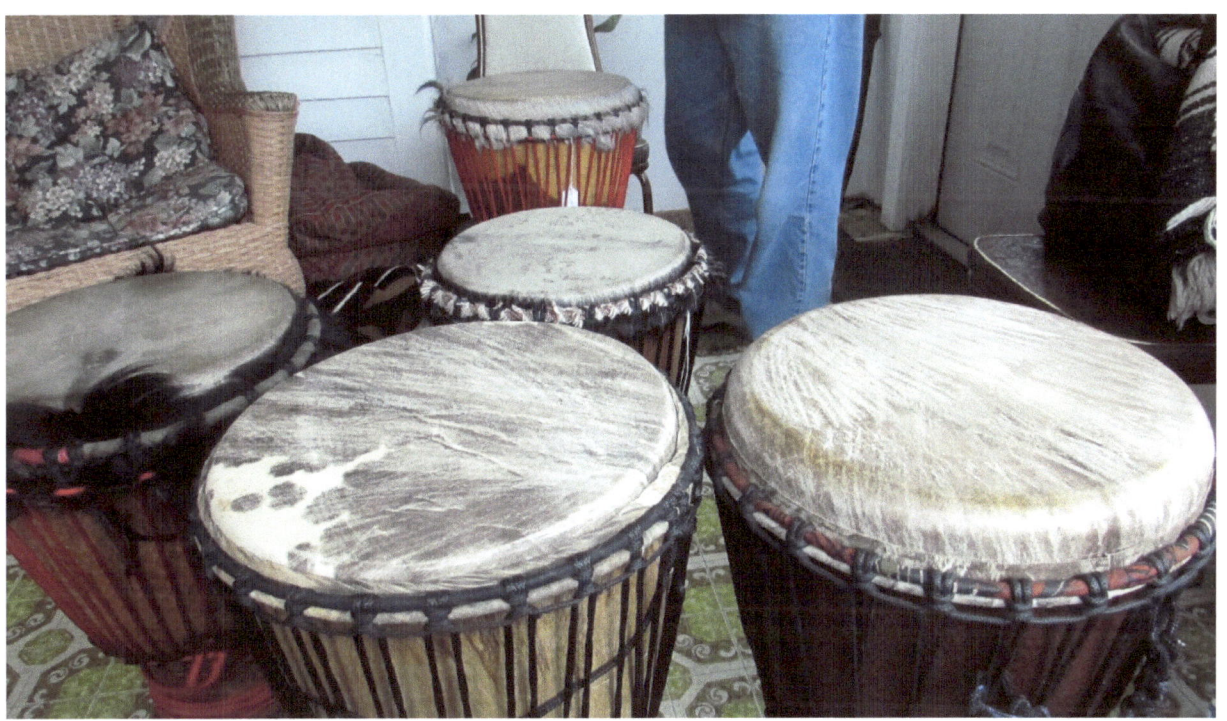

Is drumming for you? What new things would you love to try?

Looking for new ways to decrease my own stress has been a lifelong path and drumming also helps with stress reduction and balancing yourself; a drumming circle is a group activity that has meaning and purpose.

Hatha Yoga

Hatha Yoga is a form of yoga that is the art of good health and long life. Marianne Kohler wrote a book called: *The Secrets of Relaxation* where she speaks on how yoga can help you with stress and relaxation in your life. And if you need to learn how to de-stress, lower you blood pressure, lose some weight, yoga can really help.

Hatha yoga is concerned with the body and the breath. It can be of great use if you suffer from fatigue, need to manage your nerves, are hypersensitive and super-emotional, if you sleep badly or if you are looking your age!

What is Yoga?

As opposed to gym exercises, yoga is a series of movements that are slow and controlled.

Your body becomes harmonious with your mind, body and spirit.

ASANAS

The *asanas* (poses) become different masterpieces of your body like an art form. You stay in the poses effortlessly (after much practice!)

What do the postures help with?

You will find that the postures can help with rheumatism and arthritis. They massage the viscera (your belly fat), activate the bile, stimulate the intestines, liver and can even regulate your metabolism.

The 3 phases of Asanas: How the Postures Work to help you

1. When you assume the posture, your muscles work in a fashion that is slow, progressive and continuous. This becomes the dynamic phase of asana

2. The "Freeze." This is the static phase. You freeze in your chosen posture. You are transformed into a statue. You remain still for 3-4 breaths and then with practice 8-10 breaths. You can stay in asanas for as long as you feel comfortable. You are in the flow of stillness.

3. The return. Slowly you return to your original position. You relax your muscles, get back to your breath and when you are ready, another posture begins. At the end of your asanas, you should never forget to rest. This is as important to your practice as the breath and asanas.

RESTING BETWEEN ASANAS

Rest is important. Do not neglect it. This little rest time is part of the third phase. This is when nothing seems to be happening. But in Eastern thought, it is taught that the rest should be at least the same length of time as the asana preceding it.

Do Not Force things

Yoga is a practice.

In time you will get better at your practice.

Do your exercises with regularity. Ten minutes a day may be better than 1 hour a week. If you force yourself, you will be strained and your muscles will contract. True yoga should be practiced with suppleness and ease.

Pain

Stop at once if you feel any kind of tension or concentration.

Then wait a few moments. If pain persists, abandon the exercise until the next day. If pain disappears (which is more likely), push yourself and try again. But always stop at the threshold of any kind of pain.

Other conditions: If you have hypertension forward bends staying in any poses such as downward facing dog and standing straddle should not be practiced. Check with your doctor before doing any kind of exercise if you have conditions that would warrant modifying poses.

Relaxation and stress tips from: Kohler, M. (1973) *The Secrets of Relaxation.* New York, NY. Warner Communication Company

I hope that you can find your inner self in mind, body and spirit through a yoga practice as I have. *The light in me sees the light in you.* Namaste.

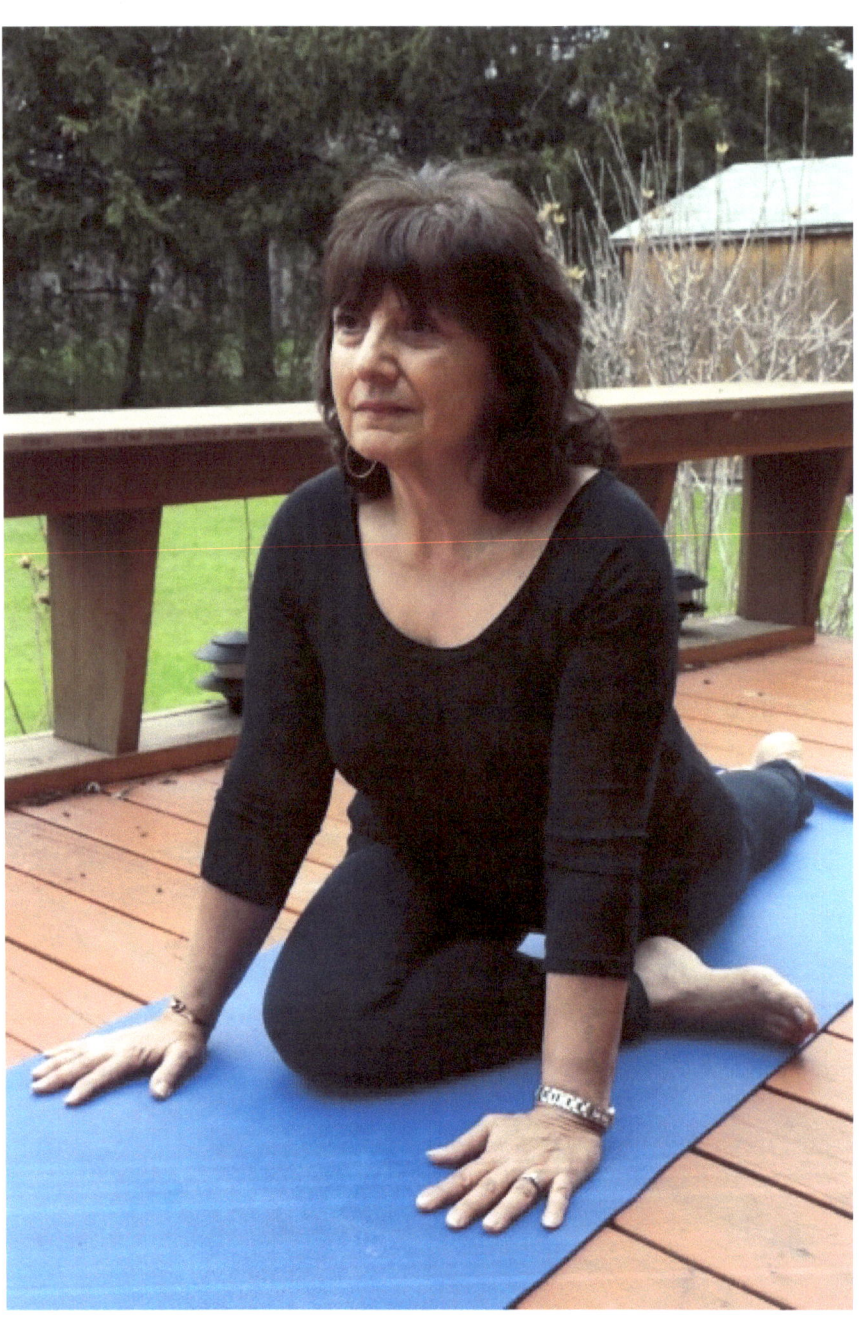